Healthy Lifestyle against Cancer

Become a Cancer Survivor, A Nutritional and Mindset Approach

1st. Edition

Amie Armstrong

<u>**Disclaimer Notice:**</u>

Please note the information contained within this document is for educational and entertainment purposes only. Every attempt has been made to provide accurate, up to date and complete, reliable information. No warranties of any kind are expressed or implied. Readers acknowledge that the author is not engaging in the rendering of legal, financial, medical or professional advice. The content of this book has been derived from various sources. Please consult a licensed professional before attempting any techniques outlined in this book.

By reading this document, the reader agrees that under no circumstances is the author responsible for any losses, direct or indirect, which are incurred as a result of the use of information contained within this document, including, but not limited to, —errors, omissions, or inaccuracies.

In loving Memory of

Maria Guadalupe
Sandoval Martínez,

Mother of 3 sons and
grandmother of 3 kids...

Table of Contents

Introduction

Cancer. It's one of those words that strikes a lot of fear into the hearts of people who have been told they have it and the people who love them. And for good reason: many people have died from cancer and have died in agony and suffering. It's one of the worst ways to leave this world and, as such, the Big C looms large and strikes much fear into the hearts of many people, even those who don't have it.

I want to tell you that cancer isn't as scary as you may think it is. While cancer is certainly an enemy that nobody should belittle or take for granted, it's not an unbeatable foe. Why should you believe me? It's because I've looked at it square in the eyes, wrestled with it and have won the battle. Yes, it wasn't an easy battle. But as hard as it can be, it can be won. And I've written this book to show you how you can beat the Big C by living a healthy lifestyle.

In this book, I'll share what cancer really is, how it develops and attacks the body, and two ways you can use a healthy lifestyle to beat the living hell out of it; prevention and treatment. Most of what I'll be sharing with you pertain to minimizing your risks of acquiring this disease because your odds of beating cancer are 100% if you're able to avoid it. And to successfully avoid it, you'll need a holistic approach, i.e., living a healthy lifestyle, which I'll share with you.

Many of the preventive lifestyle approaches can also be done to supplement cancer therapies, in case you already have cancer. That's why most of my discussion about living a healthy lifestyle as a means to overcome cancer involves these approaches. In fact, all the more reason you'll have to use these approaches if you already have cancer. Through these healthy lifestyle practices, you can supplement the efficacy of available cancer treatments, which we'll enumerate and describe in Chapter 3.

Now, if you're ready to beat this thing called the Big C, turn the page and let's begin!

Chapter 1 - Know the Enemy

The best way to beat an enemy is to know it well. That's why the battle against cancer starts in the mind by knowing the enemy. What is cancer, really?

Contrary to popular belief that cancer is a single disease, it's actually a collection of interconnected diseases. In just about any kind of cancer, some cells of the body divide uncontrollably and spread onto other tissues within the vicinity. It can begin in any part of the human body, which is made up of cells - too many to count (think trillions).

How Cancer Destroys the Body

Under normal circumstances, our body's cells grown and divide so that they can form new cells according to our body's needs. Upon aging or being damaged, cells die and, in their place, new cells are created.

This normal process is disrupted when a person has cancer. What happens during cancer is that the aged or damaged cells continue to live instead of dying a peaceful death and new cells continue to be created despite not being needed by the body. The uncontrollable growth in the number of excess cells can result in body growths we know as tumors, i.e., masses of tissue.

There are 2 kinds of tumors that form as a result of this abnormal disruption in the cellular management process; benign and malignant. Benign tumors don't multiply and spread to other surrounding tissues. However, some benign tumors can grow big. But when removed surgically, benign tumors normally don't return. While benign tumors generally aren't life-threatening, benign tumors in the brain can be.

Malignant tumors are the cancerous kind, which can multiply and spread to surrounding healthy tissues. As malignant tumors continue growing, some of their cancerous cells can separate and go to other further areas in the body via the lymphatic system or the bloodstream. When this happens, these breakaway cancer cells can create new tumors in the areas they've penetrated.

Cause and Drivers of Cancer

Specific changes in our genes can create cancer. And because it's related to genes, it's considered as a genetic disease. In particular, these changes involve how cells grow and divide. And being genetic in nature, cancer is a disease that can be passed on to us from our parents.

But cancer isn't always because of faulty genes that were passed on to us. It can also arise from DNA damage brought about by cellular division errors or lifestyle choices such as diet and environmental toxin exposures.

Every cancer patient's cancer contains a unique set of genetic changes, which can increase as his or her cancer progresses. Even in the same tumor, different cells can change in different ways. Cancer cells go through more genetic changes - like DNA mutations - compared to healthy, normal cells. In some cases, the changes don't cause the cancers but are caused by cancers.

There are 3 types of genes that are primarily affected by cancer-causing genetic changes; proto-oncogenes, DNA repair genes, and tumor suppressor genes. These genetic changes are sometimes referred to as cancer's primary drivers.

Proto-oncogenes are the genes that are responsible for managing normal growth and division of cells. But if these genes change in specific ways that make them more active than they need to be, they can become cancer-generating genes (i.e., oncogenes). And cells grow and survive even when they aren't supposed to because of oncogenes.

DNA repair genes are genes that take care of DNA that's damaged. Cells that have mutated DNA repair genes usually cause additional mutations in other genes. And when these mutations are combined, cancer cells are created.

Finally, tumor suppressor genes also play a role in managing the healthy rate of cellular growth and division. But cells inside tumor suppressor genes that are altered in certain ways can also grow and divide in unmanageable ways.

The Spread of Cancer in the Body

When cancer cells spread from one area of the body to another, it's called metastasis. This result from cancer cells breaking away from their source or origin (i.e., the primary cancer), traversing the lymphatic or circulatory system, arriving in other areas of the body, and creating new tumors (i.e., metastatic tumors) in said areas. This resulting tumor is the same kind of cancer as its parent tumor. And the cancer resulting from this type of tumor is called metastatic cancer. For example, when lung cancer spreads and has metastasized into the liver, the resulting cancer isn't called liver cancer but metastatic lung cancer.

When viewed through a microscope, you won't see any difference in the physical appearance of the metastatic and the primary cancer cells. These cancer cells normally possess the same molecular features.

Cancer treatments can help extend the lives of some metastatic cancer patients. But for the most part, metastatic cancer treatments are aimed primarily at controlling the growth of the metastatic cancer or to reduce its symptoms. Because metastatic tumors can damage a person's normal body functions severely, many people who die because of cancer usually die because of metastatic cancer instead of the primary or original cancer.

Chapter 2 - Minimizing Risks

Looking back on it now, I realized that the battle with cancer doesn't really start once a person is diagnosed with it. It starts even before a person shows symptoms or gets diagnosed with it. As cliché as it may sound, prevention is really much better than cure. It's like one's chances of surviving against a fight with Floyd Mayweather or Manny Pacquiao are 100% if one simply avoids a fight with any of these 2 great boxing warriors. With cancer, the battle begins with prevention.

Many people - myself included - think that cancer is all about the genes or one's fate. Through scientific studies, researchers have seen that it's not just genes or fate that determines whether or not one will be in an actual fight with the Big C. It's a combination of different factors, including genes, most of which we can control or influence. That means, to a great degree, we can minimize our risks of developing cancer.

Damage to DNA is the primary reason for developing cancer. Essentially, our DNA is the chemical equivalent of a drill sergeant's instructions to his trainees on what they should do. Our DNA determines how our body's cells will react to certain stimuli in our environment like the foods we eat, the sun's ultra-violet rays, stress and substances we ingest such as alcohol or nicotine in tobacco products. While the individual damages to our DNA from these factors are negligible, it's their accumulation over extended periods of time that can really start to mess up our DNA. And when the damages become too great and continue multiplying in the body, that's when cancer is born.

Going back to genes, just how much of it is really responsible for cancer? It is estimated that only 2% to 3% of cancer cases are caused primarily by poor genetics. This means that 97% of the time, cancer is caused by things that we can have a great degree of control over such as lifestyle, diet and exposure to carcinogenic substances.

How to Lower Risks of Cancer

As mentioned earlier, a great chunk of cancer cases aren't genetic in nature. This means you can do a lot of things to minimize your risks of cancer or if you already have it, optimize the efficacy of your current cancer treatment. These include:

- Minimizing or, if possible, avoiding exposure to tobacco, including second hand smoke or smoke coming from other people's cigarettes.
- Eating Healthy: In particular, you can significantly reduce your risks of cancers by minimizing consumption of red meat

and saturated fat (including trans fats), charbroiled meats, and foods that are deep-fried. You should also increase your daily consumption of cancer fighting and preventing foods such as whole grains, vegetables, and fruit, which are all abundant in dietary fiber.

- Exercising regularly.
- Maintaining a healthy body weight. Obesity is a primary risk factor for many serious ailments, including cancer.
- Limiting your alcohol consumption to 2 drinks at most daily. Excess alcohol consumption can lead to cancers of the colon, liver, esophagus, larynx, and the mouth. If your family has a history of any of these cancers, it'll be best to avoid alcoholic drinks altogether.
- Minimizing your exposures to radiation. Go for x-rays only when needed and limit your exposure to direct sunlight, especially between 10:00 a.m. to 3:00 p.m., which is when sunlight is at its hottest and most dangerous. Don't fret over the radio frequencies emitted by your gadgets and power lines - they're negligible and aren't proven to cause cancers.
- Avoiding exposure to environmental and industrial toxins like benzene, asbestos, polychlorinated biphenyls (PCB), and aromatic amines.
- Minimizing your risks of certain cancer-causing infections such as HIV, hepatitis, and HPV infections. Avoid using contaminated needles and unprotected sex to minimize such risks.

- Taking low doses of aspirin regularly. It appears that men who take non-steroidal anti-inflammatories like aspirin have lower risks of colon cancer and even prostate cancer. But if you have acidity and gastric bleeding issues, it's best to skip this.

- Getting enough Vitamin D, i.e., between 800 to 1,000 i.u. daily, which researches claim to help reduce one's risks for certain cancers like colon and prostate cancers. Get your Vitamin D primarily from food and sunlight but if you can't get enough, consider supplementing.

Chapter 3 - Cancer Treatments

If you already have cancer, the battle's not yet over. I'm telling you from experience that cancer can be defeated if diagnosed and treated in a timely manner. While it can be a rather challenging battle to fight, it's one that you can win with the right treatment, support of family and friends, and an indomitable attitude.

Thanks to modern science, there are now several ways to treat cancer, the choices being determined by the severity and type of cancer one has. Some cancer patients only need 1 type of treatment while others may require multiple treatments in combination.

Let me give you a word of caution. You will have a lot to study and think about when faced with treatment options for cancer, which means you may feel confused and overwhelmed. But let me also give you encouragement. You can feel more in control of the situation and more upbeat if you talk to your doctor and let him or her explain to you the advantages and disadvantages of each type of treatment instead of having to Google everything yourself. You can also feel stronger and more persevering if you surround yourself with family and friends who are supportive, just like I had when I was being treated for my own cancer.

Cancer treatments include:
- Surgery: The cancerous part of the body is surgically removed to stop the spread of cancer.
- Radiation Therapy: This uses high radiation doses to eliminate cancer cells and to reduce tumor sizes. Before choosing this therapy, ask your doctor about its possible side effects too, so you would know if it'll be more beneficial than detrimental to your health and quality of life.
- Chemotherapy: This type of treatment kills cancer cells via drugs. As with radiation therapy, ask your doctor about its benefits and potential side effects too before choosing to undergo chemotherapy.
- Immunotherapy: This treatment aims to strengthen your immune system to the point that it can successfully fight cancer.
- Targeted Therapy: This is a type of therapy that specifically zones in on developments in specific cancer cells that make them develop, distribute, and propagate.

- Hormone Therapy: This is a treatment specifically for prostate and breast cancers. It treats such cancers by managing or lowering hormone levels to slow down or stop the growth of such cancers. Ask your doctor about its benefits and potential side effects before choosing this therapy.

- Stem Cell Transplant: This is a cancer-treatment procedure that works by restoring blood-forming stem cells in the bodies of cancer patients, which were significantly reduced or destroyed by high amounts of radiation or chemotherapies. Ask your medical professional about its advantages and potential disadvantages so you can make a clear and informed decision whether or not to undergo this type of cancer treatment.

- Bio-Oxidative Therapy: This is a type of treatment where small amounts of hydrogen peroxide or medical ozone are introduced into a cancer patient's body to treat cancer. Doing this can help speed up the body's metabolism of oxygen and promote the discharge of oxygen atoms in the body's cells via the bloodstream. One of the main benefits of this therapy is that if done properly and together with other health-beneficial practices, it has practically no side-effects.

- Mitochondrial Therapy: This involves shutting down or mitigating the cell's mitochondria, which is believed to be vital for cancer cell growth. This therapy is based on the principle that if the mitochondria is shut down, so can cancer growth be shut down as well. And unlike poisons like cyanide, this type of therapy is able to shut the mitochondria down without damaging healthy cells. While this therapy isn't mainstream just yet, advances in studies aimed at repurposing known medicines that inhibit mitochondrial metabolism have shown and continue to show great progress and it won't be long before this type of cancer therapy becomes mainstream.

Chapter 4 - Nutrition

When it comes to cancer prevention or treatment, no single type of food or supplement can serve as a magic pill. It all boils down to your overall diet. Looking back now, I knew I could have eaten better before being diagnosed with cancer. While I can't say for sure how much of my victory over cancer has been due to changing my nutritional habits, I can definitely say that it was a major factor because I believe in the saying that "let food be thy medicine."

The Diet-Cancer Connection

Researches have shown that up to 70% of a person's lifetime risks of cancer are within one's power to control and change. And a big chunk of this 70% is nutrition or diet. It has been said that we are what we eat. I believe that - if we eat unhealthy, we become unhealthy and conversely, we become healthy when we eat healthy foods at healthy amounts.

Diet isn't just about what not to eat but about what to eat as well. While research hasn't shown solid cause-and-effect relationships between specific foods and cancer, these have shown associations between such. And part of these associations seems to include specific types of diet and low rates of cancer in certain societies.

Take for example the famous Mediterranean diet, which is rich in vegetables, fruit, and healthy dietary fats in the form of olive oil. Studies have shown that groups of people who live in the Mediterranean - particularly the Greeks - have substantially lower rates of cancer and heart disease and have associated this with how they ate. The same can be said of the people who have the highest percentage of really old people, i.e., centenarians or people 100 years or older; the Japanese. The particular area of Japan with the highest concentration of ultra-old people is called Okinawa, from where another famously healthy diet has been formed - the Okinawa diet. As with the Mediterranean diet, the Okinawa diet is also rich in heart healthy dietary fat, i.e., Omega-3 fatty acids.

Practical Ways to Implement a Cancer-Preventing Diet

To implement a diet that can help you minimize your risks of cancer or to supplement your current treatment's efficacy, most of what you eat on a regular basis must include healthy fats, whole grains, beans, nuts, and vegetables and fruits that are rich in anti-oxidants. Also, you must also minimize your consumption of deep-fried foods, processed foods, refined sugars, refined carbohydrates (white bread, etc.), and unhealthy fats (trans fats and saturated fats).

Anti-Oxidants

And speaking of eating anti-oxidant rich foods, here are interesting facts about them:

- Plant-based foods that contain abundant amounts of antioxidants can help make your immune system much stronger and help your body fight cancer cells much better;
- You can also lower your risks of esophageal cancer by eating Vitamin C-rich plant foods like dark leafy vegetables, bell peppers, peas, berries, and oranges;
- You can lower your risks of esophageal and stomach cancers by eating more non-starchy vegetables such as beans, spinach, and broccoli;
- You can lower your risks of larynx, pharynx, mouth, and lung cancers by eating more vegetables that have good amounts of carotenoids (a type of anti-oxidant) such as squash, Brussels sprouts, and carrots;

- You can lower your risks of lung and stomach cancers by eating more fruits every day; and
- You can lower your risks of prostate cancer by eating more watermelons, guava, and tomatoes - all of which are high in the anti-oxidant called lycopene.

Just how much fruit and vegetables should you eat daily? Ideally, 5 servings. And no, processed fruits and vegetables such as commercially available apple juice or carrot juice don't count. Consume mostly whole food versions of fruit and vegetables to get the most cancer-combatting nutrients while minimizing potential carcinogenic ingredients like refined sugars.

<u>Dietary Fiber</u>

Also referred to as bulk or roughage, dietary fiber is crucial for a clean and healthy digestive system. Some of the best sources of dietary fiber include whole grains, vegetables and fruit. Dietary fiber can also help lower your risks of cancer - specifically colon cancer - by allowing you to continuously move and flush carcinogenic compounds out of your digestive system via regular and healthy bowel movement.

<u>Healthy Dietary Fats</u>

It's not necessarily true that a high-fat diet can increase your risks of cancers. If the types of fat you normally consume are unhealthy ones such as saturated and trans fats, then you will be at high risk of cancer, not to mention heart disease. But with healthy dietary fat, e.g., unsaturated fats, the opposite is true.

Trans fats primarily come in the form of hydrogenated oil that's abundant in deep-fried and packaged foods like deep-fried chicken, French fries, hard taco shells, crackers, cookies, piecrusts, cakes, muffins, and pizza dough. So, if you're fond of these kinds of foods, you should radically reduce the amounts of these foods that you eat.

Saturated fat, on the other hand, comes primarily from red meat and dairy products. Your best bet is to limit consumption of these foods to only 10% of your daily caloric consumption at the maximum.

Unsaturated or healthy fats are abundant in fatty fish (tuna, salmon), nuts, olive oil, and avocados. Omega-3 fatty acids, in particular, are abundant in fish like tuna and salmon as well as in flaxseeds. Omega-3s are also known to help make the brain and heart healthier.

Refined Sugars and Refined Carbohydrates

Blood sugar spikes have been shown to increase one's risks of prostate cancer by as much as 88%. This is aside from increasing one's risk of diabetes, which is another life-threatening medical condition. And because refined sugars and carbohydrates are surefire ways to spike your blood sugar levels every time, you should minimize or if possible, eliminate your consumption of these food items. It may sound impossible, but there are practical ways you can minimize consumption of these types of foods. For example, you can substitute unrefined whole grains like brown rice, quinoa, multi-grain or whole-wheat bread, oatmeal, bran cereal, and non-starchy vegetables for refined ones like commercially available sweetened cereals (cornflakes, Cheerios, Fruit Loops, and Special K), white bread, and pasta. These unrefined grains aren't just healthier, but they're actually more filling and can give you longer-lasting energy throughout the day.

Red and Processed Meats

The link between eating a lot of red and processed meats like salami, pepperoni, sausages, and bacon, and cancer has been clearly established by numerous scientific studies. Your risks of colorectal cancer can go up by as much as 20% simply by eating 50 grams or 2 ounces of processed meat each day. The suspected ingredient of processed meats that's believed to be carcinogenic is the preservative nitrate, as well as other types of synthetic preservatives. And even if unprocessed, high red meat consumption can still increase your risks for cancer.

If you want to minimize your risks of developing cancer, minimize your consumption of red and highly processed meats. A very practical way to do this is to eat other protein-rich sources that are healthier, such as nuts, eggs, chicken, and fish.

Other Ways to Boost Your Foods Anti-Cancer Properties

Because fruit and vegetables have the highest amounts of cancer-fighting minerals and vitamins and cooking can lead to reduction of such, try to eat them raw as much as possible. With fruit, that's easy. With vegetables, consider eating them in salad form with healthy dressing.

If you do cook your vegetables, try not to cook them too much and cook them only until they turn tender. Doing so can help preserve as much of their minerals and vitamins as possible.

Before eating your fruit and vegetables, wash them with a good vegetable wash. If you don't have access to a commercially available vegetable wash, you can make your own by mixing equal parts of vinegar and water together. Soak the fruit and vegetables in the wash for up to 5 minutes before rinsing with clean water thoroughly. While it may not completely remove pesticides on the surfaces, it can wash away a great portion of it.

If you're fond of strong flavors, use immune-boosting spices and herbs like curry powder, ginger, and garlic. Others include coriander, rosemary, basil, and turmeric. Not only can they help you add a lot of flavor to your favorite dishes, they also pack a lot of cancer-fighting nutrients.

Minimizing Your Carcinogen Consumption

What makes certain types of food riskier for cancer are carcinogens, i.e., cancer-causing substances. Carcinogens can be created while food is being cooked, while it's being preserved (mostly meat preservation), or as food begins to spoil. Some of the foods that contain carcinogens are preserved, dried, and cured meats (like beef jerkies, sausages, and bacons), charred or burned pieces of meats, moldy foods, and smoked foods.

If carcinogens are your highest risk factor for cancers in food, then you should make it a priority to reduce your exposure to them. Here are some practical ways you can do that:

- Avoid cooking oil over high temperatures. Your best bet is to cook oil in low heat or via baking at 240 degrees Fahrenheit maximum, which keeps fats or oils in foods from becoming carcinogenic. Broil, steam, boil or bake your foods instead of sautéing, pan-frying, or deep-frying them.
- Lessen your barbeques. Charring or burning meats can create carcinogenic substances in your food, and overdoing a barbeque can do that. When barbequing, avoid over-doing

the meat and cook at the best temperatures, i.e., 240 degrees Fahrenheit tops.

- Store oils properly. Oils can quickly turn rancid - and carcinogenic - when they're exposed to excess air, light, and heat. So, make sure you store them in an airtight container in a dark and cool place.
- Throw away moldy and funny-smelling foods. Chances are, such kinds of foods contain a strong carcinogen called aflatoxin, which is usually found in peanuts that have become moldy. To preserve your nuts' freshness for longer, keep them in the freezer or fridge.
- Microwave food the right way. By this, I mean using waxed paper to cover food while microwaving instead of using plastic covers or wraps and to use microwave safe containers such as glass or porcelain ones.

Chapter 5 - Stress Management

Psychological stress can be a significant factor for cancer. Psychological stress is what we feel when we're under significant emotional, physical or mental pressure. While psychological stress is normal and can even be healthy from time to time, experiencing high amounts of it for extended periods of time can seriously affect our health, and one way that can happen is by increasing our risks of cancer.

We usually get stressed by routine events and daily responsibilities, as well as irregular happenings like sickness and trauma. Healthy stress - the kind that makes us better in terms of health and character - is referred to as eustress or good stress. The kinds of stress that makes us feel overwhelmed and unable to manage and control the goings-on in our lives is the bad kind of stress, i.e., distress. And science has shown that distress can be a major factor for cancer, whether in terms of acquiring it or managing it.

The Body's Stress Response

When your body experiences emotional, mental, or physical pressure, it copes by releasing producing specific stress hormones that trigger your fight-or-flight mechanism as a means by which to escape or overcome a perceived threat. These hormones include norepinephrine and epinephrine and these can help you act faster and stronger under perceived threats.

Chronic stress, i.e., long-term and high-level stress, has been shown to cause health problems such as urinary, fertility, digestive, and immune system problems. And with a weakened immune system, a person can more easily catch viral infections like colds, flu, and cough. People who suffer from chronic stress also tend to be more susceptible to anxiety, depression, insomnia, and migraines.

But it seems that these conditions don't include cancer. In which case, can psychological stress actually cause cancer? Scientific evidence linking chronic stress directly with cancer isn't conclusive. However, psychological stress can still increase one's risks of cancers but in an indirect way. How?

People who are chronically stressed tend to cope with it by acquiring specific habits or behaviors that in the long run can increase their risks of cancer. Such habits or behaviors may include alcohol drinking, overeating, and smoking, all of which increase cancer risks.

But, what about those who already have cancer? How can chronic psychological stress affect them? The stress of having cancer can be caused or exacerbated by the diseases physical, emotional, and social effects. Believe me, these can really stress you out and make you do unhealthier things that can lower one's quality of life during and even after cancer treatment.

But chronic stress shouldn't defeat you. I was blessed to have family, friends, and church members who helped me manage my psychological stress and, as a result, I was able to respond much better to cancer treatments and have since been able to live a good quality of life. Some of the benefits of learning how to manage one's stress while battling cancer include less cancer-treatment related symptoms, less anxiety, and less depression. In terms of cancer survival, however, stress management has no scientifically established benefits. But still, it can help you cope better with the disease, which can improve your quality of life and in some indirect ways, your chances of survival.

How I Coped with Stress

I experienced the great benefits of getting a lot of social and emotional support during the cancer treatment stage of my life. It has kept me from becoming depressed, greatly reduced my initial worries about being diagnosed with the Big C, and has significantly reduced symptoms related to both the cancer and the treatment. In particular, I learned to cope with stress during that difficult stage of my life through talk therapy, meditation, relaxation practices, joining a support group of cancer patients and survivors, and regular exercise.

But for me, the single biggest thing you can do to manage stress well is to surround yourself with family and friends. Cancer isn't a battle you can win alone - you'll need the strength, support, and love of others to carry you through the disease's most challenging stages. If not for family, friends, and my church, I probably would have gone bonkers because of my cancer. But thanks to them, I didn't. Not only did I manage to keep sane but I managed to slug it out and win the battle against the Big C.

Chapter 6 - Regular Exercise

As mentioned earlier, 70% of cancer risk factors are within our ability to control or manage. And most of the 70% are lifestyle choices. One of them is getting regular exercise, which is one of the best things you can do to minimize your risks of cancer. And if you already have it, I can tell you that it was one of the best habits I have acquired that have helped me improve the quality of my life even while I was going through cancer treatments.

Think about this: it's been estimated that about 33.33% or a third of deaths due to cancer were because of sedentary lifestyles and obesity. And these deaths include two of the most prevalent types of cancers in the United States: colon and breast cancers. By exercising regularly, you can avoid a sedentary lifestyle and in the process, minimize your chances of becoming obese.

How Much Exercise?

Based on national activity guidelines, exercising for a minimum of 30 minutes daily for most days of the week, i.e., at least 4 days weekly, is a good place to start. And if you'd like to optimize the health benefits of regular exercise, exercising for 60 minutes daily is a good goal to aim for.

What about the type of exercise? Should you do CrossFit, weights, sprints, swimming, etc.? At the minimum, you should do moderate-intensity exercises like brisk walking or jogging. But how do you estimate intensity? You can use the "talk test" to do so.

Here's how the talk test is done. While you're exercising, try to talk as if you're carrying on a conversation with a friend. If you can talk normally as if you and your friend are just catching up in a coffee shop, your exercise intensity is light. If you can hardly talk and are gasping for breath to just to say something, that's high intensity. If you can still carry a normal conversation, but with some breathing strain, then that's moderate or mid intensity.

How do you adjust exercise intensity? If you're doing aerobic or cardiovascular exercises such as brisk walking, running, swimming, or biking, you can do so by increasing the speed at which you're performing the exercise. You can bring the intensity level down by slowing the speed at which you're doing the movements. If you're lifting weights or doing resistance training exercises like calisthenics or suspension training (think TRX), you can increase intensity by increasing the amount of the resistance or slowing down the movement. To reduce intensity, reduce the amount of resistance or upping the speed of movement (momentum makes it easier to work against resistance).

To optimize your regular exercise experience, you can consider doing the following too:

- If you don't have enough stamina to complete a 30-minute exercise session yet, you can break it down into 2 15-minute sessions or 3 10-minute sessions within the day;
- To minimize your risks of dying from boredom with your aerobic or cardio workouts, listen to your favorite music or exercise with a friend;
- Drink lots of water and dress in comfortable clothing during your workouts; and
- Respect your body. If you're not feeling well or are running a fever, don't exercise. Rest and give yourself time to get well.

Other Practical Ways to Exercise More Regularly

If you don't have enough time or energy for the exercises I mentioned above, it doesn't mean you can't exercise anymore. It's not an all-or-nothing proposition. Getting some form of exercise - even if it's below the minimum - is much better than not getting any at all. Here are other practical ways that can help you exercise more regularly:

- After every meal, walk around the block once or twice;
- Dance at home or if you can, join a class;
- Ditch the elevator and use the stairs instead;
- Instead of commuting to or riding a car or bus to your destination, try to walk or bike instead;
- Instead of e-mailing or texting your co-workers or classmates, walk up to them and talk to them directly instead;

- Park at the farthest possible spot from your school, office, or wherever you're going to so you can walk the farthest distance possible;
- Walk as much as you can during the day and aim for at least 8,000 steps daily, which you can measure using a pedometer-equipped app or device like Fitbit; and
- While watching T.V., do something active like ride a stationary bike or perform planks or crunches.
- You can clean the house or tend to your garden - they can be very good workouts too, especially if you do them for over an hour;
- Tai chi and yoga are 2 good alternatives for regular exercise as they incorporate meditation (good for stress management) and movement;
- If you're already undergoing treatment for cancer and are unsure of what types of exercises you should go for, consider checking out exercise programs that are specifically designed for cancer patients, which are available in some hospitals and health centers; and
- If you're currently going through radiation therapy, don't swim for exercise because doing so chlorine can irritate your radiated skin and because your immune system may be weakened during radiation therapy, you may easily catch an infection in the water.

Conclusion

Thanks for buying this book. I hope that through this book, you were able to learn and be encouraged that cancer - while it's a formidable foe - can be beaten! But more importantly, I hope that through this book, you were encouraged to take action by applying what you learned here. Remember, knowing is just half the battle and the other half is action or in this case, application of knowledge. You don't have to apply everything you've learned at once. Just apply one lesson at a time. The important thing is you start acting on the information you've gleaned in this book and do it soon. Cancer isn't an opponent that takes kindly to procrastination. Cancer is a swift opponent and if you want to beat it, you'll have to be just as swift, if not swifter.

Here's to your victory versus cancer! Cheers!

References:

1. https://www.cancer.gov/about-cancer/understanding/what-is-cancer
2. https://www.cancerresearchuk.org/about-cancer/causes-of-cancer/can-cancer-be-prevented
3. https://www.health.harvard.edu/newsletter_article/The-10-commandments-of-cancer-prevention
4. https://www.helpguide.org/articles/diets/cancer-prevention-diet.htm
5. https://www.cancer.gov/about-cancer/coping/feelings/stress-fact-sheet
6. https://www.cancer.gov/about-cancer/treatment/types
7. https://www.alive.com/health/bio-oxidative-therapies-the-power-of-oxygen/
8. https://www.cancer.gov/research/key-initiatives/ras/ras-central/blog/2017/targeting-mitochondria